ABBI'S WAY

A Simple, Effective Way of Eating that Results in Weight Loss and a Lifetime of Weight Management

ABBI'S WAY

A Simple, Effective Way of Eating that Results in Weight Loss and a Lifetime of Weight Management

BY ABBI L. BAYERSDORFER

ARTSMART PUBLICATIONS

TAMPA

Abbi's Way:

A Simple, Effective Way of Eating that Results in Weight Loss and a Lifetime of Weight Management

ISBN 978-1548235116

The information and reference guides in this booklet are intended solely for the general information for the reader. The contents of this book are not intended to offer personal medical advice, diagnose health problems or for treatment purposes. It is not a substitute for medical care provided by a licensed and qualified health professional. Please consult your health care provider for any advice about your health or before starting any diet, exercise or supplementation program.

Contents

Dedication

This book is dedicated to my sister, Jill Baldarelli, who sadly passed away, earlier this year, of heart failure. She loved both cooking and her family dearly.

For our family, food is synonymous with love. A few weeks before her passing, she experienced that love in the form of sharing our family's homemade ravioli's (ingredients include a special meat, spinach, romano cheese and a nutmeg/lemon rind filling, with homemade sauce, courtesy of my sister-in-law, Catherine).

After my sister's funeral, her friends and family were able to eat her homemade raviolis one last time. I swear I heard Jill say, while I was eating them - "Well, at least Ab, you got to have some rav's today, because you missed them at Christmas."

I love you, Jill, and miss you, your love, humor and food, a lot. This book is for you, as well as, all those who want to be in charge of their body instead of being the adverse effect of it. In other words, to those who want to be their own "food boss" and are willing to say, "no" to the "must do" diet defeats.

You are my inspiration for this book and I thank you from the bottom of my heart!

Acknowledgements

We have so much to teach one another. I have learned from so many in my lifetime. I can recall being in the kitchen, as a little girl, with my mother, learning her recipes that had been passed from generation to generation. I considered myself very fortunate to have received those gifts.

This book would not be possible if I hadn't learned from some great teachers how to correctly eat and effectively control weight. This work includes what I have learned from them which I codified into what I know is a workable and fun way of eating and controlling weight.

I would like to personally thank those I have learned innumerable lessons from in my lifetime:

- My mother, Mary Baldarelli
- Nutritionist, Adele Davis
- Award-Winning Executive Chef Zoltan
- My brothers and sisters
- My husband
- My daughter
- The dedicated clients of Abbi's Way

Foreword
By Dr. Steve Ryland

"The doctor of the future will give no medicine, but will instruct his patients in care of the human frame, in diet and in the cause and prevention of disease."

– Thomas A. Edison

Having been in the medical profession, for over 20 years, and seeing my patients, family, friends and our community getting sicker, at younger ages (including many close friends who are no longer with us), the above words mean so much to me.

Here are some facts:

- One out of two men and one out of three women will have cancer in their lifetime
- One out of three people are considered obese
- 33% of the population will be diabetic by the year 2050
- One out of three people are suffering from heart disease, the silent killer

Currently, we don't have a healthcare system; we have a disease management system. When you become sick, the system is there to manage your disease.

The fact is over 70% of all diseases are preventable; I repeat, over 70% of all diseases are preventable. So prevention is the key. The truth is prevention is better than a cure as this old proverb states:

"It's easier to stop something happening in the first place than to repair the damage after it has happened."

So how do we prevent our bodies from breaking down and getting sick? The solution is much simpler than you might think.

Let's take a car for example. If you change the oil periodically, put gasoline in the tank, rotate and balance the tires, and perform other general maintenance actions, the car is going to have a longer life span. In other words, there is less chance of it breaking down than the car that doesn't receive the same care and maintenance.

The same can be said of our bodies. If we perform general maintenance, fill our "tank" with proper nutrition, get plenty of sleep and reduce stress, our bodies will reward us with a happier, healthier and more productive life span.

Eighty percent of our battle comes in the form of our diet. You are, indeed, what you eat!

The pages you're about to read will change your life, for the better, in so many positive ways. I have known Abbi for years and I applaud her intention, willingness, knowledge and professionalism in advancing a solution in living a far healthier life.

It is with great pleasure and admiration that I introduce you to "Abbi's Way". Frankly, this program works naturally and is as necessary as the oxygen we breathe.

I wish you the very best of health!

Introduction

Observing my husband and myself slowly putting on weight after countless attempts at diets was, to say the least, disheartening. Experiencing the ups and downs of dieting and the struggle that ensued to maintain our weight was, to put it mildly, frustrating. As the holidays were fast approaching, I knew something needed to be done but the thought of getting on another diet...ugh! The old adage about doing the same thing and expecting different results was staring me in the face once again.

Were we really going to experience the hardship of another diet?

Were we really going to set ourselves up for feeling the excitement of losing weight and then the apathy of gaining it all back again, months later?

Then one evening, I noticed my husband short of breath and showing pain in his chest, while he was sitting in our room. Important to note, my husband was 289 pounds - the heaviest he had ever been. He was only 45 years old and his body changed significantly since being that stud, All-American athlete, in college, at 225 pounds.

At the moment I saw him in pain, I thought...

I could be spending the rest of my life as a single mother without the man I love dearly. So I made a very firm decision:

We were going to change his physical condition fast. Come hell or high water, he was going to get healthy fast and I was going to ensure it happens now!

It was amazing to experience the results of this simple but powerful decision. I learned to trust my basic knowingness on the subject of food and eating, no matter what the latest fad diet said to do. I observed my own results, my husbands results and my clients results and I write this book from those observations.

I spent too long believing someone else, because of their education level and popularity, knew more than I did or ever could about dieting, weight loss and weight management. That is until I tried many, many different diets, lost weight and gained it back over and over again. Having confidence in my abilities and myself, I decided I could find a way out of the "yo-yo diet" mess that left us wanting for a simple program based on truths that worked.

YOUR
RESULTS

CHAPTER ONE

YOUR RESULTS

Some schools of thought say, if you lose weight too fast, you won't be able to maintain the weight loss. Moreover, that you should only have a 2 lb. weight loss, per month, so you can maintain your weight. This idea is a falsehood. It is an example of the innumerable false ideas and "diet must do's" that exist out there about losing weight.

Simply stated...

Results are what help you persist on a given course. Get no results and winning doesn't occur. Get results and the winning keeps you going.

We live in a world, with the common reality, that results need to happen fast. More often than not, the expectations that all the intended results will happen overnight bring about disappointment and dismay. That is not how results come about physically. Results happen, step by step, over a period of planned time.   They can be as fast or as slow as you agree to experience the results.

Your attitude and thoughts about losing weight, and maintaining your weight, are the driving force of Abbi's Way. If you believe you're too old to lose weight; your metabolism is too slow; it will take a long time to lose weight; you can't maintain your weight loss, etc., you will experience all those barriers. Come hell or high water, you will find a way to make yourself "right" about not losing weight. However, if you change your attitude about losing weight and keeping it off, you will persist, find what works, and win from here on out.

Here is a list of the results my husband experienced over a brief period of time:

Week 1 –
- On the fourth day, he said he had a lot more energy waking up
- By the sixth day, he said he could see, hear and smell more clearly
- By the seventh day, he felt more aware and could solve problems faster
- Within 7 days, he lost 11 pounds

Week 2 –
- He observed he could focus his attention for longer periods of time
- He no longer was getting impatient
- He said he was sleeping much more deeply and feeling consistently well-rested
- The back pain he had been experiencing for years started to subside
- He lost another 6 pounds

Week 3 –
- He noticed his skin looked healthier
- His waistline was 2 inches less
- His clothes were starting to feel baggy on him
- He lost another 6 pounds

Week 4 –
- He lost another inch on his waistline
- He said he felt as if his body was healing itself from years of abusing it with bad food and loads of sugar
- He was sleeping soundly every night
- He smiled more often and was overall feeling very happy about various parts of his life
- By the end of week 4, he lost another 9 pounds for a total of 32 pounds lost, since he started Abbi's Way

Other Client Results –

One for one, the clients who have done my program say...

- They had more energy within the first week
- Their energy increased as they continued onward with the program
- They were not hungry doing the program (a "diet
first" for all of them)
- They felt like doing some form of exercise and did so after being on the program (important to note – you don't have to exercise to lose weight on Abbi's Way)
- They are amazed they could maintain their weight after losing it

The results you'll get will be your results. It is important to look for them and acknowledge them. Write them down in the spaces provided in The Abbi's Way Workbook and keep them close at hand so you can read them often. Validating your wins is an important part of this program.

Don't ever put your attention on feeling badly about not losing weight.

Find out what you did or didn't do and fix it for next time. There is always a next time. Don't be sad, apathetic and depressed about it; be interested and stay in action.

A helpful tip is to review your successful actions and find out what you did that made you successful and do that again.

If you run into trouble, at anytime during this program, please go to Chapter 6 Persist Despite All Odds. Reviewing this chapter will help you with the needed encouragement to keep going and reaching your intended goals.

THE
PROGRAM
DEVELOPMENT

CHAPTER TWO

THE PROGRAM DEVELOPMENT

My husband and I tried many types of diets over the years and some were good and some not so good.

We had tried the 500-calorie diet with the female hormone, about 3 times in the last 5 years, and each time it did work. But each time we gained the weight back. It was also harder and harder to do since the hormone became regulated to the point where it was difficult to get the drops over-the-counter. Not to mention, the fact that my husband, deep down inside, wondered if he was going to grow breasts or act like a "girl", taking the female hormone.

Then we tried the synthetic and natural supplement

drops, while doing the diet. They were the same price as the actual drops but didn't seem to work at curbing the appetite in the same way. This 500-calorie a day diet just was not enough food for me and definitely not for my husband, with or without appetite curbing or fat burning drops. We were hungry, irritable, fought a lot and pretty much turned into Mr. and Mrs. Jekyll and Hyde for the entire weight loss part of the diet.

Granted, it was not that long of a diet (21 days), and wow, you can lose 1 to 2 lbs. a day! Those are some amazing results and the reason why my husband and I went on the diet, or anyone in their right mind, would go on such a diet for that matter. But it was still way too long for our liking, let alone, our household and our marriage. When your daughter asks you, "Why are you mad all the time, Mommy?" Ouch! There has got to be a better way to get results. So I posed a question:

Do we really need to take hormone drops or any other weight loss aide to successfully lose weight and keep it off? I concluded - **No, we don't, and Abbi's Way of eating was born**.

Another similar question came to mind:

Can you still have that kind of weight loss and eat enough food so you don't feel like you're going to pass out or kill someone? Abbi's Way Answer - a resounding, YES!

So moving on, my husband and I tried the diets where you had to count calories and stay within a calorie range to lose weight. Yes, that worked...for a day! I apologize to all those people who like doing this horrible, tedious task. But by my very nature, I'm not a calorie counting, weigh-my-food-before-every-meal kind of gal. As far as I'm concerned, there's not enough time in the day for this process. Even with all the nutritional info you can find on the Internet, it just isn't worth it.

Having to do another "calorie counting", "portion weighing" diet just makes me want to do a sit-in on my kitchen floor, not budging an inch, protesting to the very end, waiting and ready for the Bulldozer of Diet Must Do's to run me over.

What about those diets that give you a set amount of food that comes by mail or a set portion or a set number of calories that is the same for every man, woman and child on earth? You eat one meal and it leaves you wanting more. I could easily eat, and sometimes did eat, 3 or 4 of them, at one sitting - a serving size made, by old Grinchy Clause. A meal that was even too small for the other Who's mouthses! I don't' know about you but I like to eat a good size portion of food, diet or no diet.

Next question:

Do you really have to count calories and measure out every morsel of food to lose weight? Abbi's Way Answer – No, you do not!

How freeing is that? That just freed up, like half of your day right there, for other really fun stuff or at least things that don't make you want to tear your eyes out.

So how do you get away with not counting calories or weighing your portions? By eating the right type of weight-loss-producing foods.

Let's take a look at the very simple basics about losing weight – The Law of Input vs. Output. We know it, we've heard it, it's proven that if you eat more food than your body needs to sustain itself, it will be stored as fat. Not new news. If you burn more calories than you consume, you will lose weight. Yes, a very simple and well-known principle that can be very hard to follow.

I found out a secret. You can eat a lot of the right types of foods, which will give you lots of energy. By staying in, just under the input amount of calories that is right for you (explained in the first stage of the diet), you will feel great and lose weight. You don't have to starve yourself. You actually eat a lot more food during the weight loss stage than on the maintenance part of Abbi's Way! It's hard to believe but you can eat twice as much of the weight loss foods - good whole foods, energy producing foods and not be hungry, while losing the intended weight.

So we were well on our way to doing Abbi's Way! Without pills, drops or weight loss aides and the hardship of not eating enough food to sustain our bodies and keep conscious. The best part – we lost weight, we felt really good, slept well and were very healthy doing it.

The next question:

Do you have to exercise to lose weight? With Abbi's Way, it is not required that you exercise.

I know this statement is going against just about every diet and weight loss book ever written. We all know the benefits of exercise. It is proven to help you feel better, look better and lose weight, keeping in mind The Input vs. Output Law. I remember after I had my daughter, I peaked during my pregnancy at 200 lbs. I like to be around 128-130, which I am now, while writing this book. Even with running, after I had the baby, I didn't really lose the baby weight. I got frustrated and thought...what the hell am I doing all of this running for and still not losing weight? I know now that I was not eating the right foods and eating more than I was burning, violating the law.

What happens on the days, weeks or months that you can't go out and give yourself a walk or regular exercise? Do you just give up on losing weight entirely? I hear too many people say, "I know I should go for a walk or a run or go to the gym, but I'm too tired, I don't have enough energy". Just the thought of having to get up early before work or after work, when you are dog-tired, and go do a workout? Nope, not gonna happen!

Well, a funny thing happens around the 2nd or 3rd week of doing Abbi's Way. You actually feel like going for a walk or a run or doing something that resembles some form of exercise. It's an amazing side effect of the program. It happens, that by starting to lose weight, that bad knee, that had too much weight on it before, doesn't hurt so much now when you walk. Or the jiggling that you feel is a little bit less, and you're not as self-conscious about moving that body around. For instance, my husband started dancing again when we went out. And he can bust a move with the best of them!
In conclusion, you don't have to exercise to lose weight but we all know the benefits.

Again, one for one, my clients, on their own self-determinism, started exercising because they now had the energy to do so and they felt even better.

An important note about exercising on the program:

Your appetite will increase in proportion to how much exercise you do.

Good news - you can eat more! The bad news –
there's a tendency to overeat when increasing your
exercise level. Therefore, I chose very light exercise,
while in the weight loss stage, so I did not risk
overeating.

With Abbi's way, moderate to heavy exercise is
better done during the last two stages of the diet.
But again, weight loss can still be accomplished with
diet alone.

THE BILLION-DOLLAR QUESTION

CHAPTER THREE

THE BILLION-DOLLAR QUESTION

Have you ever been on a diet and the urge to cheat was overwhelming and overpowering, so much so, that you didn't just cheat a little bit, but you downright had a freak out, binge session? One that made you feel, not only physically sick but emotionally like you just shot your best friend's cat? Right, pretty bad, so you know what I'm referring to - that horrible experience of dieting and cheating and letting yourself down and going through all of the self invalidation that takes place to the point where you just give up entirely on your diet and yourself. How can you fix that problem of dieting?

Doing Abbi's Way of eating, with enough food, prevents that starving, deprivation feeling. You feel like you ate enough and are full.

So that is one plus-point but there is another plus-point to this diet. A plus-point is actually putting it mildly here, let's just call it for what it really is, shall we...

It's a full on, Christmas Morning-Santa came and left you lots of everything you wanted under the tree and your stocking is brimming over with abundance plus-points.

Hence, the most important billion-dollar question:

*Could we incorporate a "cheat day" once a week that would make it okay and not the evil, immoral, devastatingly debased and damning thing that it normally is to cheat on your diet? Abbi's Way conclusion number three – **YES WE CAN!***

God, that felt good to write that and even better to have it! The chains of past diet deprivation and can't have diets just flew off and broke into a million, billion pieces.

Yes you can, once a week, have a "cheat day" and eat whatever you want. It's a total slap in the face of the word, "diet" because diet implies that you can't have things that you're restricting yourself, and limiting what you have. By the way, the actual derivation of the word diet comes from the Greek, "diaita", meaning a way of life. That's what it should mean - a way of life and eating that makes sense in this crazy, GMO, fast food, chemical world.

Now there is no way that I am going to profess and tell you that incorporating a cheat day, once a week, in a diet would give you the same results as not cheating. That's very hard to do. But it can increase leptin hormone levels, fool the body into thinking it is not on a diet, and also rev up the metabolism once a week.

Emotionally, I will say that it did wonders and amazing things to our attitude about losing and maintaining our weight. Just the thought of a cheat day coming up in the near future, once every week, made life on a diet livable again. Dreaming and imagining all the wondrous tastes and sensations of the Willy Wonka Experience to come, made doing the weight loss stage of Abbi's Way actually workable and might I add, fun.
How many diets can you say are fun?

So then a funny thing happens when you incorporate such a crazy and infamous day. When that day comes, every 7 days, sort of in a biblical way, something shy of incredible happens. All the things you wanted to eat, supersizing yourself silly with treats and sweets and falling into Wonka's Chocolate River of bliss didn't actually happen for me, for my husband or my clients. It was a startling change. We could eat anything we wanted. Anything, and yet it wasn't that fun to cheat like we had done before on other diets. We were loosing weight rapidly, feeling really good, and cheating with various foods we desired. But we found ourselves cheating in a good way. Eating healthy, saturated, fatty meats, cheeses and, yes, we had some wine and nuts. It was like a Roman holiday for us; just those items were enough to satisfy. I will confess that on that first cheat day, I had a handful of Halloween candy and some dessert but it wasn't what you might think it would be.

What I would plan on doing naturally was to arrange the upcoming parties, as it was during the holidays, around the cheat day. I would naturally tend to eat less on that day like other types of calorie-conscious diets. I would eat less during the day and then eat what I wanted at the party and I found that even when I tried, I couldn't really eat all that much. It was really cool. Then when it came time to cheat the next week it was naturally healthier and healthier choices. Not because I had to but because I wanted to and it brought me back to being cause over those cheat days. Not the effect of the uncontrolled sick binge thing that would take place on other diets. I could choose exactly what I wanted to eat and face the consequences of those food choices.

Would I add more time to my diet by consuming way over the calories allotted for weight loss? Would I give myself a sugar headache the next day for overdoing it? Sometimes yes because I was going to have some birthday cake at my daughters' friend's party and other times I was winning too much on the diet to do that and I chose the healthier cheat food items. Sometimes it would be just one dessert I was craving like chocolate lava cake and that was enough. Other times it was all about the carbs and I would eat pasta and savor it. It certainly wasn't stale bread. It was warm, fresh out of the oven French bread, with real butter, and that was fantastic. So yes, go ahead, have a cheat day once a week. But you decide what foods and how much weight will be gained the next day.

So what actually is taking place here?

You regain control over what you eat. The binge doesn't rue (ruin) you; you rule the day!

*Notes and precautions on the once a week Cheat Day:

If you already have a medical condition like diabetes, an autoimmune disorder or a heart condition that you are on a special diet for, you will need to consult your doctor to see what foods you can incorporate into your cheat day. I am not stating here that if you're diabetic that it's okay to go on a candy binge or if you are a cardiac patient that you can eat hamburgers and fries on your cheat day. Absolutely not! You need to get a food list from your doctor to see what are the allowable cheat day foods and work closely with a health professional.

As for the rest of us, the cheat day will depend largely on what type of results you want to get on the diet. How healthy you want to make it and what foods are right for you. Will you cheat with good fats or bad? Will you eat avocados or fries? It will be up to you.

When I was doing the weight loss stage of Abbi's Way, the cheat days were more important to me than when I started to maintain my weight and incorporate other types of foods. It was around the holidays and it seemed every weekend there was another holiday party. I would see which party I wanted to have my cheat day on and for the first time had no guilt at the party. I was excited about attending, (unlike some parties, where I dreaded going because of all of the tempting foods I couldn't have that would stare at me, commanding me to eat them.) That was a bit crazy, the food was telling me to eat it instead of making my own decision about what I was going to eat.

So then going to the parties, I noticed another amazing thing. I looked around at the beautifully decorated rooms, amazing smells, and wonderful holiday treats and the incredible thing was that I could have everything I wanted in the whole room! I could have the whole holiday party experience really for the first time!

Then I would run into friends and talk to people and we would mosey on up to the food stations and more than one person would tell me how they couldn't have whatever it was on the table.

"Oh look at that, incredible dessert, I would love to have some of that, but no, I can't have that, I had to give that up" with a sad, forlorn kind of look on their face.

And what was I thinking at the time? You poor

bastard, I was like you once. But I can eat anything in this room that I want and I proceeded to do just that!

In reality, I found that I didn't actually eat everything in the room, I had a little piece of this and tried some of that and it was so much fun. No guilt or inner struggle. I actually enjoyed talking to people again at parties (or maybe for the first time as this inner struggle with food was going on for a long time). I didn't realize how much attention I had on the food soap opera that was happening within me. I would miss out on whole conversations with people. Gone was the distracting conversation I would have with myself that went something like...

"Should I eat that, no, don't do that, oh but I really want some of that, I know but you really can't eat that, and you said you wouldn't, yes I know, but I want to have it, but no you really shouldn't...."

Then of course I would give in to that inner food devil and I'm surprised the host didn't check my purse for valuables because I acted like I just stole their gold plated dish soap dispenser out of the bathroom. I definitely couldn't concentrate on anything anyone was saying because I was ready to bolt out the door for fear that my inner food demon, just unleashed, and would precede to wipe out the entire buffet.

So yes, there was something profound about this cheat day. I started listening to other people and enjoying myself at parties. That was a big win for me. I hope it helps you, too.

THE BIG FAT DEBATE

CHAPTER FOUR

THE BIG FAT DEBATE

To eat fat, or not to eat fat, that is the question:

Whether 'tis nobler in the mind to suffer the slings and arrows of the low fat, high carb and sugar diet, or to take arms against a sea of diet related diseases, and by opposing them, eat a lot of saturated fat?

And then what? In another 50 years, we will find out that eating too much good fat is still bad for you! I don't know about you but I don't have another 50 years to find this out.

You don't have to be a scientist to observe a diet high in carbohydrates and sugar can make you fat. High fat, high protein diets were the solution to this and are not new. They have been around for many years and include diets high in good fats and protein and low in refined carbs and sugar.

I tried many of the high fat, high protein diets and, yes, they were better than the low fat, high carb and sugar diets. But over time, as it is very easy to over consume good fats, I gained weight. I was 20 lbs overweight doing a high fat, high protein diet. Then I got a body fat scale and was shocked to find out that my % body fat was in an obese range for my age. Granted, I did eat good fats. So was I full of good fat or bad fat? At 20 lbs overweight, I didn't really feel the need to find out if my LDL's (a type of cholesterol) were fluffy or sticky. I just wanted to lose weight and have good nutrition doing it (if you want to know if you have good or bad cholesterol, see a healthcare professional).

You can lose weight and still have high body fat.

It's not the amount of weight you have but the amount of body fat that's potentially dangerous to your health.

Carrying too much body fat can increase your risk of developing serious health problems such as high blood pressure, high cholesterol, heart disease, diabetes and cancer. Maintaining a healthy, body fat percentage can reduce your risk and help prevent the onset of these conditions. That's why in Abbi's Way, you measure overall weight and % body fat to make sure you're losing both. There are some scales that measure total weight, % body fat, water weight, muscle mass and bone density. That's great to have all of those measurements, but the two main statistics that I track are:

1. Overall weight
2. % body fat

Especially, as you get close to reaching your ideal weight. You will notice that you start to register less weight loss overall but will continue to lose body fat and see a decrease in your measurements and clothing size.

So what is the simplicity with the fat frenzy? That you can be overweight and unhealthy, with a high level of bad cholesterol and sticky LDL's, possibly have hardened plaque-filled-arteries, and at risk for diabetes, heart disease, stroke and even cancer. Or be overweight, filled with good fats, and possibly at a lower risk for diet-related diseases. Either way, you'll want to lose weight.

In addition, you can lose weight by eating really healthy, organic whole foods, or you can lose weight by eating pesticide-ridden fruits and veggies. It depends on how healthy you want to do it.

The Abbi's Way of eating is:

A whole food eating plan, with nutrient-rich-lean-proteins, as well as, low carb veggies and low glycemic fruits which provides great nutrition for the body. This program satisfies hunger, revs metabolism and burns fat the natural way.

It is not a no fat diet! Why am I suggesting, in the face of now popular public opinion, that you should eat less good fat, more protein and veggies and low sugar fruits to lose weight? Because it works and you feel good... that's why!

We have to go back to The Law of Input vs. Output. Fat has almost double the calories of protein - 1 gram of fat, good or bad, has 9 calories compared to 1 gram of lean protein, which has 4 calories. I would rather eat a lot of protein and veggies that will give me sustained energy than go around drinking coffee and grass fed butter all day. You need protein and veggies for your body's nutrition, not fat and coffee. Protein suppresses hunger better than fat. It takes longer to leave your stomach than fat so you feel fuller, longer. You will have more energy by eating lean protein and veggies as compared to the same amount of good fat, or bad, for that matter.

Proteins take work to digest, metabolize and use, so you will burn lots of calories processing them. They give you the nutrition needed to build and repair all kinds of tissues, muscles, hair, skin and organs. Enzymes, antibodies and hormones all depend on proteins and amino acids to build lean muscle. Muscle burns fat.

In comparison, fat tissue burns about two calories per pound, per day. While muscle tissue of the same weight burns seven calories per day. That is the whole point of losing weight, right? Burning fat! I would rather burn up what extra fat I have than eat a lot of good fats and have to burn up those before I even get to burn stored fat, good or bad. With Abbi's Way Diet, you're still getting the recommended 20-30% of good fats each day.

A note about reaching ketosis, which is a metabolic state in which the body burns fat as a primary fuel source - you can reach this state on Abbi's Way. You will need to modify your cheat day to exclude carbs and sugar.

I know I reached this state while doing other high fat, low carb diets. There is only one little thing – The Law of Input vs. Output. I gained weight even though I was in a state of ketosis and I'm sure I was in a healthier state overall but still 20 lbs. overweight. I found it too easy to overeat and consume more calories than I burned on the high fat diets. Abbi's Way diet uses good fats, contained in proteins and veggies. You are more than welcome to add more good fats, if you desire. I do include more good fats in the other stages and on my cheat days. But you'll have to reduce your portion size, during the weight loss stage one, and weigh yourself to make sure you're not gaining weight and body fat. There are many ways to lose weight; I found Abbi's Way to be the fastest, healthiest, and most fun way to do so.

THE STAGES OF ABBI'S WAY

CHAPTER FIVE

THE STAGES OF ABBI'S WAY

To sum up Abbi's Way, it has three important stages:

> Stage One - Weight Loss
> Stage Two – Weight Maintenance
> Stage Three - Cheat Days

In Stage Three, the cheat day will be very different from person to person. For example, my brother Richard, who is an avid cyclist, has a carb cycling day for his cheat day and eats sweet potatoes and high carb legumes and whole grains, packed with nutritional value and calories. He also chooses to substitute lean animal protein for a plant-based protein several times a week to aid in his nutritional journey.

The Abbi's Way of eating can be adapted to any eating style:

1. Ketogenic (fat metabolism)
2. Paleo (cave man diet- where you eat meats, fish, nuts, leafy greens, regional veggies and seeds, etc.)
3. The Autoimmune Protocol (which is a stricter Paleo diet, involving the elimination of grains, legumes, dairy and processed foods)
4. Vegetarian (no meat)
5. Vegan (no dairy and no meat)
6. Gluten-Free (no wheat)

There are many variations of the above but those are the general diets of today. *Again, Abbi's Way can be applied to all of them with excellent results.*

In Stage One, here is the vital data you need, to start losing weight:

- Eat and drink, the allowable foods and drinks, on the program for 6 days, with the 7th day a cheat day
- Take weight and % body fat in the mornings, after going to the bathroom, before eating and drinking
- Then after successfully losing weight for 2 weeks, weigh in once a week on morning of the cheat day

- Whenever new foods are introduced, weigh in each morning
- Determine, from stats, what the next week's program will be
- If lost 4lbs or more, continue same actions
- If under 4lbs lost, figure out what needs to be changed
- Two meals per day or 3 meals, with one shake
- Two snacks of fruit and egg whites
- Xylitol or Spry gum in between meals. Drink plenty of fluids
- Tablespoon of milk or non-diary per day in coffee or tea
- Water, coffee and tea
- No sugar drinks. Add Stevia or can drink Stevia soda or sparkling flavored waters like La Croix

The meat and veggies of the diet and the calorie amount will vary from person to person. As well as, with women and men, your size and how much you need to eat to feel satisfied each day.

Rule of thumb: One part protein to two or three parts veggies.

I used 6 ounces of lean protein for me; 8 ounces for my husband, per serving, and used an assortment of low carb veggies for each of the two meals. This is a start and you determine how much protein is right for you as you progress.

My husband ate his bigger meal in the morning, with more protein, and a lighter amount of protein at lunch. He had little to no dinner, and occasionally a piece of fruit. I, on the other hand, ate my first meal at lunch and second at dinner and had fewer portions than he did. I used egg whites and would cook two-dozen eggs in the beginning of the week to have on hand.

For those people who require three meals a day, you can poach egg whites in broth and add veggies for a simple breakfast. Or, I have had success with my diet coaching clients, by having them use a protein shake for breakfast that is low glycemic and nutritious. Keep in mind, The Law of Input vs. Output and eat a lighter meal for dinner (before 6 PM).

So here are the weight loss foods on Abbi's Way Stage One (another rule of thumb – organic and natural is best):

- Tea or coffee in any quantity

- Sugar free natural sodas like Zevia or La Croix (natural flavored sparkling water)

- Only one tablespoonful of milk or natural non-dairy allowed in 24 hours

- Natural, no calorie sweetener Stevia or Truvia.

- Drink plenty of water - ½ gallon, minimum per day, if possible. Each of your two meals include (breakfast and lunch or lunch and dinner)

Protein:

- 6 to 8 ounces of veal, beef, chicken breast, fresh white fish, lobster, crab or shrimp. This is a guideline to start. You may need less or more to lose weight or to feel satisfied
- All visible fat must be carefully removed before cooking
- It must be boiled, grilled or baked without additional fat
- 4-5 containers, fat free chicken, beef or bone broth
- The chicken breast must be off the bone
- Canned tuna packed in water
- 1 or 2 egg whites with each meal or as a snack between meals

- Poach egg whites in non-stick pan with a few inches of chicken, beef or bone broth
- No oils, butter, or any other fats used in cooking

Vegetables:

- Spinach, chard, chicory, beet-greens, green salad, tomatoes, celery, fennel, onions, red radishes, cucumbers, asparagus, cabbage, and brussel sprouts
- Can have any combination of vegetables with protein

Fruit:

- A large apple, strawberries, blackberries, one grapefruit or one large orange
- Put Stevia and real vanilla extract on fruit for more flavor

Seasonings:

- Fat free, sugar free, carb free natural spices, red wine or apple cider vinegar, lemon, hot sauce, fresh and dried garlic. Any fresh or dried herbs

- Sugar free and oil free natural extracts like vanilla

A typical week for me in Stage One would be to take a trip to Trader Joe's. You can buy organic and natural foods much cheaper there than most other places.

<u>Meal Plan Examples:</u>

Breakfast, lunch and two snacks or lunch and dinner (not eaten after 6pm) and two snacks

Meals pick two - breakfast and lunch or lunch and dinner:

Salads:
- Handful of lean protein, chicken or eye of the round lean beef, cooked as specified below
- Can mix two kinds of protein if you like

Seafood:
- White fish, shrimp or crab legs, no butter or fat

Dressing:

- White or red wine or apple cider vinegar mixed with water and flavored with Stevia, salt and pepper, fresh herbs or dried herbs and spices
- I like cilantro, or thyme. Whatever you prefer
- Grey Poupon mustard with hot sauce or mild salsa

Here is some great cooking advice from my dear friend, Chef Z, who is an award-winning executive chef that will make your Stage One meals a true culinary experience...

"Cooking is a craft and an art. To play music, you have to know each key on the piano. Imagine that these keys are the spices in cooking. You have to decide what styles you want to play depending on your personal liking. Choose the spices that you know first and then do little experiments with other new and interesting ones. Remember before you go too extreme that you are the one who will eat it!

"Is that fun?

"Oh yes, it is! Taste the melody that you created. We have to focus on having fun, and play the game of how to cook, without fat.

"Everyone has a unique flavor profile that he or she likes. The recipes are guidelines to one's way to do what he or she likes. If you know the guidelines and items, you can create your own dishes, so you can eat exactly what you like so you'll look forward to each meal and forget that you have to eat with restrictions. The focus will be on what you can have, not what you can't."

He recommends the following cooking methods:

1. Broiling - dry heat from above.
2. Baking - dry heat in oven.
3. Boiling - immerged fully in liquid.
4. Braising - cooked in short liquid, covered.
5. Poaching - cooked in simmering liquid.

Additional Info...

- Wrapping - use baking paper or banana leaf
- Crock Pot - for stews and casseroles, or 'one pot' dishes
- Non-stick pans are used to "sear" or "sauté"
- Cooking vegetables in short liquid and then puree in the blender and add some of the

cooking liquid to it. This is the way to make purees

- Vegetables to use - lettuce (any kind), cabbage, kale, chard, onion (any kind), tomatoes (any kind), asparagus, cucumber, fennel, radishes, celery and brussel sprouts
- Proteins to use - no bone, take skin off and trim the fat
- White fish, lobster, shrimp, crab, chicken, beef (attention on fat%, it has to be lean)
- Fruit to use - apples, blue-black & strawberries, grapefruit, oranges, lemons and limes
- Use aromatic herbs to flavor
- Use chicken breast due to being the lowest in fat
- Trim all the fat off beef, then cook it. For ground beef, use the 96% premium lean
- If you tenderize meats, it will be thinner and the cooking time shorter so less chance to dry out.
- When you cook it in a non-stick pan, put your favorite spices on it, then rub it in, put into the hot pan and cook both side 3-4 min depend on the thickness of the meat.

You can use for seasoning: Worcestershire & mustard, Braggs Liquid Amino & ginger, smoked paprika, granulated onion, granulated garlic, rosemary, thyme, basil, chive, parsley, cayenne pepper, Tabasco, apple cider vinegar or any natural herb or spice.

Your meal can be done in a short time, with preps 30-40 min. Serve it with salad made from the above vegetables. Below are the spices and blends for different cuisines. The spice group will be yours to select and create for your own taste. Put your name on it! You can do your own blend, with a small coffee grinder.

Cajun & Creole Spices:

Allspice, basil, bay leaves, black pepper, caraway seeds, cardamom, cayenne, celery seed, chives, chile peppers, cinnamon, cloves, cumin, dill seed, dill weed, garlic, gumbo filé, lemon, mace, marjoram, nutmeg, onion, oregano (Mediterranean), paprika, parsley, saffron, savory, tarragon, thyme, white pepper and yellow mustard.

Blends: Blackened Seasoning, Cajun Seasoning, Cajun Turkey Rub, Creole Seasoning and Cajun Rub (hot), Mesquite Seasoning.

Caribbean Spices:

Allspice, achiote seeds (annatto seeds), black pepper, chile peppers, cinnamon, cloves, garlic, ginger, lime, mace, nutmeg, onion and thyme .

Blends: Adobo Lime Rub, Caribbean Spice, Caribbean Turkey Rub, Colombo Powder (Caribbean curry powder), Jamaican Jerk and Mojo Seasoning.

Chinese Spices:

Cinnamon, cloves, fennel seed, ginger, hot mustard, lemongrass, Sichuan peppercorns, star anise, Tien Tsin chiles, turmeric and white pepper.

Blends: Chinese Five Spice.

Indian Spices:

Anise seed, ajwain, asafoetida, bay leaf, black cardamom, black cumin, black mustard seed, black pepper, black salt, brown mustard seed, chile peppers, cinnamon, cloves, coriander, cubeb berries, cumin, dried mango, fennel seed, fenugreek leaves, fenugreek seeds, garlic, ginger, green cardamom, lemon, lime, long pepper, mace, mint, nigella, nutmeg, onion, poppy seeds, saffron, sesame seed, star anise, turmeric and white pepper.

Blends: Garam Masala, Panch Phoron, Madras Curry, Maharajah Curry, Vindaloo Curry and Tikka Masala.

Italian Spices:

Basil, garlic, onion, oregano (Mediterranean), marjoram and parsley.

Blends: Italian Seasoning, Pizza Seasoning, Spaghetti Seasoning and Tuscany Bread Dipping.

Mediterranean Spices:

Basil, bay leaves, black caraway, black pepper, cardamom, chervil, chile peppers, chives, cilantro, cinnamon, cloves, coriander, cumin, fennel seed, fenugreek seeds, garlic, ginger, juniper, mace, marjoram, mint, nutmeg, onion, oregano (Mediterranean), paprika, parsley, rosemary, saffron, sage, savory, tarragon, thyme, turmeric and white pepper.

Blends: Citrus Seasoning, Greek Seasoning, Herbs de Provence and Mediterranean Dry Rub.

Mexican Spices:

Allspice, achiote seeds (annatto seeds), basil, Mexican cinnamon, cayenne, chile peppers, cilantro, coriander, cumin, epazote, mint, nutmeg, oregano (Mexican), sage and thyme.

Blends: Adobo Seasoning, Habanero Mango, Manzanillo Seasoning, Mole Seasoning, Taco Seasoning and Yucatan Recado Rojo.

Middle Eastern Spices:

Aleppo pepper, anise seed, caraway, cardamom, cumin, maras pepper, nutmeg, sumac and turmeric.

Blends: Baharat, Lebanese 7 Spice, Shawarma and Za'atar.

North African Spices:

Birds eye chiles, cilantro, cinnamon, cubeb berries, cumin, garlic, ginger, grains of paradise, long peppe, mint, onion and saffron.

Blends: Baharat, Berbere, Harissa, Moroccan Chicken Spice Rub, Moroccan Vegetable Rub, Piri Piri Seasoning, Ras el Hanout and Tunisian Five Spice.

Spanish Spices:

Basil, bay leaf, cayenne, cinnamon, cloves, garlic, mint, nutmeg, oregano (Mediterranean), paprika (smoked sweet), parsley, rosemary, saffron, sage, tarragon, thyme and vanilla.

Blends: Paella Seasoning.

Thai Spices:

Basil, black pepper, cardamom, chile peppers, cilantro, cinnamon, cloves, cumin, garlic, ginger, lemongrass, lime, mace, mint, nutmeg, shallots, turmeric and white pepper.

Blends: Spicy Thai Seasoning, Thai Curry Seasoning.

Note about some seasonings:

I found that I could squeeze fresh garlic on my meals and not have the smelly problems that I normally would have when I combined fresh garlic with carbs and sugar meals. I found that I could digest it easily and wouldn't burp it up or have gas when I ate garlic with protein and veggies.

Baked Chicken Recipe:

- Take fat free chicken breasts, and cut any remaining fat
- Place in baking dish, season both sides with
    - Dried Minced Garlic go to spice
    - Salt and Pepper
    - Fresh Lemon
- Bake 350 degrees for 1 hour, flip side after ½ hour until thermometer reaches 165 degrees
- Put ¼ inch of chicken broth on bottom of pan

Crock Pot or Clay Pot Roast Beef:

- Go to butcher of your local grocery store and ask them to cut you a 2 or 3 lb. eye of the round roast and trim all fat off. Season as desired
- Place in crock-pot, with ½ inch of fat free chicken or beef broth.
- Cook for 6 hours on high or 8 hours on low setting

- I use the drippings, after cooking, to season my soups or anything else needing more flavor

Season well:
- Salt, pepper
- Dried minced garlic
- Soy sauce
- Vinegar (not balsamic)
- One Stevia packet
- Fresh onions
- Fresh celery
- Alterations:
- Drop of liquid smoke (not the healthiest but tastes good!)
- Nutmeg
- Lemon

Eye of the Round Steak:

- Pound into submission
- Marinate with red wine vinegar
- Magic Blackened Steak Seasoning
- Dried minced garlic
- Salt and pepper
- One packet of Stevia

Fish, Shrimp & Crab Legs:

- Broil with lemon and garlic, Blackened Redfish Magic spice. Add diced tomato with basil and garlic over top
- Boil shellfish in lemon, Old Bay Seasoning, bay leaves, minced or garlic powder
- No butter (but you knew that)

Shrimp Cocktail:

- Horseradish
- Puréed stewed tomatoes and stevia
- Or no sugar salsa

Soup Variation:

Chicken Tortilla Soup (minus the tortilla)

- Cook chicken breasts as above earlier to have on hand (makes 4 servings)
- One onion, chopped
- Two cloves garlic, chopped
- One can (14 oz) whole peeled tomatoes
- One tbsp. chipotle pepper (no sugar or carbs added)

- Six cups chicken broth
- ¾ lb. boneless, skinless chicken breasts
- Salt and black pepper to taste
- Juice of 2 limes
- Hot sauce (optional)
- Chopped onion, sliced radishes and fresh cilantro (optional)

Directions:

- In dry pan without oil or fat, place onion, garlic and use two tbsps. or more of chicken drippings from above, sauté onion and garlic until soft, do not burn
- Transfer to soup pot
- Add can tomatoes, chipotle pepper
- Chicken broth
- Simmer
- Add lime juice
- Taste for salt and pepper, add if needed
- Get empty serving bowl, add handful of chicken, last ingredients if you like them
- Pour hot soup into bowl- enjoy!

Marinades:

- Let marinate overnight, if you have time
- Poor an inch of fat free chicken, beef or bone broth, right before you cook meat to make drippings to save for flavor in other meals.

All Purpose Rub:

- 1 packet Stevia
- 1 tsp. ground cumin
- 1 tbs minced garlic
- 1 tsp. salt
- 1 tsp. pepper
- 1 tsp. onion powder
- 1/8th tsp. cayenne pepper

Poultry Rub:

- 1 tbsp. chopped fresh thyme
- 2 tsps. chopped fresh sage
- 1 tsps. chopped fresh rosemary
- 1-1/2 tsps. sea salt

- 1/2 tsp. cracked black pepper
- 1 tsp. paprika

Seafood Rub:

- 2 tbsps. paprika
- 1 tsp cracked black or white pepper
- 1 tsp minced garlic
- 1/4 tsps. dry mustard
- 1 1/2 tsps. sea salt
- 2 tsps. chopped fresh dill
- 1-1/2 tsps. chopped fresh tarragon
- 1 tsp. fresh lemon zest

Steak Rub:

- 1 tbsp. chopped garlic
- 1 tbsp. chopped shallot
- 1 tsp mustard seed
- 1 tsp fennel seed
- 2 tsps. peppercorns
- 1 tbsp. kosher salt

- Blackened chicken, dry not cooked in fats, on top of a garden salad
- No cheese or croutons, no dressing
- Red wine or white or apple cider vinegar on the side
- Ask for hot sauce if you like
- I carry around packs of Sweet Leaf Stevia wherever I go to add to vinegar and unsweetened ice tea with lemon
- Broiled fish, cooked w/out oils or fats. Add to it lemon, garlic and spices (Magic Blackened Redfish spice is common)
- Pick one or two cooked vegetables, no fats.

I have had success at a pizza place, ordering a salad and grilled chicken, no fat, with vinegar on the side. I put my Stevia in the container and dilute with water. Usually, they have shakers of Italian spices and garlic powder on hand.

Salad Bar Option:

Pick salad and veggies allowed on program.
Dressing: If vinegar looks pink, it is red wine

vinegar; if it looks dark, it's balsamic, don't use that. Dill pickles are a nice option as well.

Lifesaver: Xylitol or Spry Gum! Have it on hand and eat between meals if out, especially if someone is eating food you want, so you don't cheat!

Morning meal for my husband:

- Stew meat, with cut up tomato and two egg whites, one grapefruit
- Season with stevia and vanilla extract, fresh lemon and spices
- Trader Joe's Unsweetened Tea
- Supplements and Vitamins

Morning meal for me:

Poach 2 or 3 egg whites in 2 inches of broth in a non-stick pan. Add spices, minced garlic and soy sauce. Use slotted spoon to take out egg and reserve liquid. Add fresh spinach and spices, wilt spinach and add in a chopped up tomato.

Lunch:

Soup - chicken soup with drippings from baked chicken and chicken broth, celery, minced garlic, onion six ounces of cut up chicken (or the amount that is right for you). Put in a mixture of veggies you like.

Apple salad, cut up with stevia and lemon juice. My husband would eat Spry or Xylitol gum in between meals or save fruit till the end of day.

Special Sunday Meal:

Snow Crab Legs with Asparagus, cooked with lots of lemon and garlic. Fresh cut up tomato

Get more meal ideas from the web. Eat what you like. You can do this. You won't be hungry.   And dream of the cheat day.

Weigh yourself every day to start. Adjust the amounts of protein and food accordingly, eat less if you're not losing the weight you want. Eat more if you feel weak or tired.

Thinking ahead and planning ahead will make this stage much easier. Making meals for the week and changing things up, each week, made it more interesting. Getting a thermos to take soup, on the go, made things easier to bring my Stage One food with me if I was not eating at home for lunch.

Dinner was easier to cook at home or warm up if I prepared meals ahead. Bring your Stage One foods with you and don't get stuck out without the foods you can eat so you can stay on the program and experience the many wins.

Stage Two – Weight Maintenance

This is the real crux of the diet, where the pedal hits the metal and the rubber meets the road. How many times have you lost weight and have been really excited and then didn't know how to maintain your weight? What are you supposed to do now? The major problem with stopping a diet is the inevitable weight gain. It is too easy to go over the input vs. output ratio and be unable to maintain your weight loss after dieting.

One diet we tried had a plan when you gain more than two pounds in a day it advises you to do a "steak day" and eat nothing all day and have a huge steak and an apple for dinner. This resets your metabolism and you drop the weight. I found my self doing regular "steak days" and buying steak a lot made it a pretty expensive way for me to maintain my weight.

Then I tried the high good fat diets that are so popular now. I basically accepted the fact that I just can't eat carbs and sugar, *ever again*. I limited and restricted myself to "no carbs, no sugar" and I won't gain any weight. Right? Wrong! I had a little bit more success with these diets and knew I was eating really healthy foods - healthy cholesterol and healthy fats - but still, slowly gained the weight back with an *obese body fat ratio* to boot.

How can you incorporate starches and sugars, and not gain weight? Unless you are an athlete or a young person with a very high metabolism, old folks like us who do little to moderate exercise, do not burn up the introduction of the starches and sugars on a regular basis.

It's time to think differently about maintaining your weight. This word, "maintain" is not exactly correct. You never will stay at exactly the same weight, perfectly forever. It is not realistic and trying to maintain the exact weight, day in and day out, could very well be the problem.

Let's look at what can happen after you finish your diet. You are excited and very happy at first, high fiving around in your skinny jeans and the world is a funner, happier place. And then you gain a few pounds. You say to yourself...oh well, that's okay,

I'm up a few pounds, not to worry. A week later, you're up a few more pounds and again, no biggie, right? I'll just exercise the weight off. So that doesn't work, okay, now what? I'll just eat really healthy, all Paleo, gluten free. Still not working, but I'm eating so healthy! Finally, with 10 lbs. gained you say screw it all! Why am I eating so healthily and still can't maintain my weight? I've given up lots of the foods I love and I still can't do this? Where are the chips, burn the skinny jeans and gimme the ice cream! If I'm going to gain it all back, no matter what I do, at least I'm gonna have fun doing it!

I don't know about you but I feel like we are label happy here in the U.S. We are so quick to allow others to label us and then we agree to limit ourselves and our abilities by accepting those labels.

It seems once you're labeled with something, you can't ever change it, that you're stuck with it and it's limitations.   Please see the last chapter of this book because it's not true.

So why, in my right mind, do I want to go around and accept eating-style-labels, that now limit me into one type of eating, and exclude all other kinds of food? Unless of course, I have been diagnosed with a disease, which, thank God, I have not. Therefore, I profess to - no-food-style-label. I will not go around calling myself any kind of self-imposed eating style or food label. The ketogenic diet was developed for epilepsy, the gluten free diet was developed for celiac disease, lactose intolerant means you do not produce enough of the enzyme, lactase to digest milk products. Vegan is one step beyond vegetarian and the autoimmune protocol takes Paleo to a whole new place.

Thank God for these eating styles, as they have saved lives and helped people handle and live, with the now over 80 different types of autoimmune diseases.

These eating styles are very healthy and if you look closely you will see they all fit in one or more of the 3 stages of the Abbi's Way Diet.

There's just one little thing...

I want to be able to eat the foods I want and not voluntarily label myself a certain food style, excluding all other types of food. I like carbs and sugar, so do many people. The Standard American Diet tastes good. I know it's bad for you but do I have to give all of that up forever?

I don't regret many things, except the time I was on the ketogenic diet trying to lose weight yet again. It was during Thanksgiving and I was visiting my brother and family in New England. My brother, Bert, is an amazing cook, and every year, on Thanksgiving night, he makes a meal passed down generations in my family called Turkey Soup with homemade pasta. And I, trying to reach the state of ketosis, passed up the chance to eat this soup, of the gods, that my brother slaved all day to make for us. I ate the broth and turkey. But I passed on the homemade, very thin, melt-in-your-mouth noodles that soaked up all the turkey soup broth goodness. And I missed all the fun of getting a little soup on my face, after you slurp up the last of the noodle, on your fork. In my family, food is love.

*Although my bowl was gluten free, Paleo and did not compromise my ketogenic, fat burning state, it also had a little less fun and a lot less love in it. Is it really humanly possible to maintain your weight after dieting? Finally, a resounding **YES!***

Possibly, for the very first time, you can maintain your weight loss and eat the things you want. This should be called the can-have-diet.

It's interesting that when you exclude the

problematic, highly processed carbs, sugar and even dairy for a majority of the week, and then eat them, once or twice a week, they may be less of a problem. Yes, they still may be bad for you but you might not have developed the allergy, intolerance, weight gain or problem with the food in the first place if you didn't eat it all the time. The Standard American Diet is not good for you, we know that, but I still want to eat pizza and ice cream, chocolate and petite fours. Chocolate lava cake and turkey dinner with stuffing, mashed potatoes with gravy, my mother's lasagna and yes homemade turkey soup, romano cheese with pasta en casa. You do not have to give up, forever, foods you love to lose weight or maintain your weight.

What about the cheat day? Can you still have one of those? Another YES you can.

Not only can you have one cheat day, you can have more than one and maintain your diet. Once you have reached this high condition of health and weight loss, you can afford to have more than just one cheat day. My husband and I usually just take the weekend to enjoy ourselves and eat what we want. I usually make a traditional comfort food meal that I grew up on. Like roast beef with mashed potatoes and gravy or one of my mom's Italian favorites. Or just go out to eat and splurge and have the fresh bread, dinner and dessert, like you do used to do in life.

*How is this even possible? I can't cheat one day without gaining 10 lbs., you say? This is done very simply by a workable balancing act between the three stages of Abbi's Way that allows the incorporations of **All** of the kinds of foods you like to eat in one week.*

The majority of the time you will be eating typical maintenance, healthy foods.

Once you have lost all the weight you want, you can now go ahead and eat a full on Paleo diet, or one of the many "good fat" diets that are out there now. Do add in good fats, low carbs, natural sugars, nuts and dairy. But because you are already very close to an ideal calorie intake, with the protein and veggies, you won't be adding as much of these foods to your diet to maintain your weight. You can add more of the heralded and all important good saturated fats to your diet like butter, olive, coconut oils, nuts, avocados and other kinds of good fats and foods. But your portion size will inevitably come down so you will not exceed the normal calorie intake for you to maintain your weight loss. Remember The Law

.put vs. Output and continue eating nutrient-rich protein and vegetables.

Try the addition of low carb alternatives into your diet, like baking with almond meal and coconut flours. Turn now to low carb and low sugar meals. Introduce natural starches and sugars but keeping the diet organic, natural and moderate. I especially like Paleo and autoimmune protocol diets for Stage Two Maintenance. Frequent a place like Kara Lynn's Kitchen if you live or are visiting the Tampa Bay area.

I have several of my clients who have graduated to the Abbi's Way Maintenance stage and are very much enjoying her incredibly tasty, and healthy foods that reduce inflammation (no night shades) while providing great nutrient-rich meals for the body, with the correct portion size so you won't gain weight. Your scale will be your best friend. Just as in during the weight loss stage, you need to use a scale that shows % body fat, so you can continue to track % body fat and weight. In the maintenance stage you can add in good starches and sugars, whole grains and fats all in moderation and small amounts, then weigh yourself to see if you gained weight.

So what, exactly, happens in this Stage Two-Weight Maintenance, if you gain weight? You just drop back into Abbi's Way Stage One – Weight Loss.

It's just the way it is, you know you can lose weight by eating that way, so go back to the successful action, but don't wait until you have gained 10 lbs. to drop back into losing the weight. Go back to Weight loss Stage One for as long as it takes you to re-lose the weight and stabilize again. This will only be for a few days and you still are eating really well and shouldn't be hungry. Then, adjust accordingly as you incorporate more foods.

If you did gain, take out the additional item and save it for the cheat day. Or eat less of that type of food to maintain. Use the worksheets and pages provided in the Abbi's Way Workbook or your own notebook to record the foods you start to add into your diet on this stage.

I would start to add things in slowly and one at a time so you can track what food and what amounts you added and if you gained weight or not. This is also a great way to see what foods are giving you a problem and which ones you can eat without any adverse reactions.

and that when I had the foods that normally gave me trouble, once a week, instead of every day, I could eat them and I was no worse for the ware. I realized, I do better eating dairy only on the weekends, for example, and switched to almond milk during the week and indulged in cream in my coffee on the weekends.

What does a typical week look like on the Abbi's Way Maintenance Stage? A typical week looks like this...

I now have lost all the weight I want. I've reached my target weight loss! Yea! You just won the lottery, all apples on the slot machine because you can afford to have not one but at least two cheat days! You deserve it; go for it! Then after your cheat day or days, Stage Three, you immediately drop into the Abbi's Way Stage One - Weight Loss eating plan for the next day and for however many days it takes to make sure that you lose the weight.

Once you have lost the weight, you now eat a healthier diet, incorporating good, saturated fats and healthy foods. Then, plan on a cheat day on the weekend.

What you eat on your cheat days will determine

your eating habits for the next several days. Some people may have already got the hang of incorporating food into Stage Two to the point where they don't even need to do a cheat day, Stage Three. Others may choose to stay in the Stage One for most of the week, adding in only very little fats, sugars and starches so they can go all out on their cheat days in Stage Three. This is the simplicity and the flexibility of the Abbi's Way of eating. Use common sense and be cause over what foods you will cheat with, instead of letting the foods control you.

If that doesn't work, that's okay, you have your Abbi's Way Stage One to handle it. Be happy and know that you never have to label yourself unless you want to. I actually welcomed the simplicity and healthful eating of the weight loss Stage One. After the cheat day or days, you will notice a weight gain but then in a few days you will lose again. If you don't want to gain very much, you will cheat less. It's that simple. Don't complicate it.

During the Weight Loss Stage One, I choose not to weigh myself every day for that reason. I knew I would probably not lose weight or even gain weight after my cheat day. But I also knew that I would lose that weight in the next few days and overall I lost between 3 and 5 pounds each week. I was happy with that. My husband chose to weigh himself every day and see the effects of the cheat day. It inspired him to cheat less and then he could see it actually didn't really affect his overall weight loss, and it was not such a big deal.

The less you cheat, the faster you will lose the weight. Make it a game, dream about all the things you can have and then see what you will actually eat. I would buy foods specifically for my cheat days like Trader Joe's Chocolate Lava Cake. For cheat days in Stage One, adjust your food intake, eat less to get ready for the cheat day, and then weigh yourself accordingly the next morning after the cheat day. For example fasting in the morning for a big Thanksgiving meal at night. Then recording what the weight gain was the next day. Cheat days in Stage Two, same thing and drop into Stage One the next day and subsequent days if you gained any weight on your cheat day.

An example of the Abbi's Way in action - we were on the diet over Christmas. I decided that I was going to cheat over Christmas break. We were going up to see my husband's family in North Carolina and I decided to cheat on Christmas Eve and Christmas. But when we got there that plan kinda went south and I ended up with four full-on cheat days, instead of two. Eating every manner of Christmas delight, from cookies to pies to chocolate Santa's galore. I didn't worry about it and I didn't weigh myself when I got home for fear of getting depressed. I just got right back on the Abbi's Way Weight Loss Stage One from Monday to Friday. So five days of eating really well and losing weight. I weighed in on that Friday after Christmas 1 pound and ½ % body fat less than when I went away for Christmas vacation!

Who can say they lost weight over Christmas and enjoyed themselves? It was so much fun to look good and feel good, seeing the family and not have to tell them that I can't eat the traditional, homemade, holiday offerings. Or that I was on a diet and I had to refuse some specially baked item because I was now and forever more, gluten free. No, I went away armed with papaya enzymes and probiotics and ate what I wanted to eat. Then came back home, didn't starve myself at all, just ate the weight loss foods in Stage One and I was back at my ideal weight in five days!

The way to maintain your weight is, if at any time you are gaining weight, drop into Stage One and figure out what you did that caused the weight gain, and then change it.

So going forward will be a balancing act of all three stages of eating well and the correct amounts in Stage One and Stage Two and eating the "bad foods" only once or a few times a week in Stage Three. Instead of on a regular basis.

It's a checks and balance game that you will be playing to maintain your weight for the rest of your life.

But have fun, make exciting healthy recipes, try new foods, search the Internet for nutrition-packed foods. Try new meals and make old favorites in a new healthy way. But always use your scale and drop into Stage One if you need to.

*Note, if you have more than 40 pounds to lose, you can decide to drop into the Abbi's Way Maintenance Stage for a week, each month, to give yourself a break from the diet. Then get back into the weekly weight loss. Or some of my clients have chosen to do a Stage Three cheat week and then get right back on the program with a renewed zest for losing weight.

*Notes on alcohol, sugar, carbs and bad fats. I treated these items like Stage Three cheat day food. Once you hit Stage Two Maintenance, you should use these in moderation as with any high calorie food item. Keep good records in a notebook or the Abbi's Way Workbook, and if you choose to add them more often, see if it is affecting your weight. You may need to restrict the consumption in order to maintain your weight and health.

Additional Nutritional Supplements:

There are many vitamins and supplements out there today. These were the ones we used that helped us. They are not necessary to losing weight but help with nutrition and detoxing the system, which does have a positive effect on health and weight loss.

- *JuicePlus+
- Probiotic
- Cal/Mag
- Multi Vitamin
- Digestive enzymes papaya for cheat days
- Omega 3 supplement

*JuicePlus+ is the one company I've decided to partner with after I experienced the results of the product for myself. I also saw spectacular results with my husband and clients. If interested go to - http://abbi1.juiceplus.com/us/en

However, no supplements are necessary for weight loss. If you do decide to take them, make sure they are backed by medical research and have time honored, proven results.

PERSIST DESPITE ALL ODDS

CHAPTER SIX

PERSIST DESPITE ALL ODDS

If you didn't have barriers to overcome, it wouldn't be the game called life. And it would be boring to do this program. So know that there are going to be barriers. They are just there for you to overcome. There are ways to beat them all. Just keep the frame of mind that anything can be overcome and anything can be fixed if you don't do it right the first time.

I hear my husband tell our 9 year-old-daughter often – "Anything can be fixed, Tegan". If you asked her, "What does Daddy say?" She will tell you without hesitation, "anything can be fixed!"

So don't waste time worrying or contemplating a barrier you didn't overcome yet. Just persist and all the odds will be beaten.

For instance, my husband still loves sugar but instead substitutes it with Spry or Xylitol gum. He chews as much of it as he wants. He takes Truvia or Stevia in his tea or coffee. This helps him overcome his urge to have sugar. He also takes Juice+ as a wholefood supplement to curb his sugar cravings, etc. He often drank CalMag to help him relax his nervous system. He took digestive enzymes and probiotics to help his digestive system. And occasionally he took multi-vitamins to help his entire system along with all the changes happening rapidly.

Other things he did to keep beating barriers:

He weighed himself every day. He adjusted the amounts of protein and food accordingly. He would eat less if he was n't losing what he wanted. And he would eat more if he felt weak and/or tired.

I recommend a good scale that shows % body fat. Some days during Stage One, you may not see a change of weight but you will see a change of % body fat. You are still losing, even if your weight doesn't change, your size sure will. *He would validate these wins often.*

Another way of beating the barriers is using a notebook or my workbook that aligns with this book. Here is where you can keep track of what you're eating, especially in Stage Two, Maintenance, when you need to record what you added and what your weight is the next day. After two to three weeks, you'll have a very good idea of what foods you can add and how much you can eat to maintain. Then it should be easy to know what foods and amounts help you maintain your weight and those you need to leave for the cheat days. Use these records and refer to them later as needed.

Please don't hesitate to contact me with any questions or assistance, especially if you feel the odds are winning against you. My team offers diet coaching and we are always willing to help you achieve your goals rapidly!

THE DECISION

CHAPTER SEVEN

THE DECISION

I have learned that the condition of one's body is monitored by one's thoughts. Think you will never lose weight, and you never will. Think you're starting another diet that won't work, and it won't.

However, think it will work, and continue to think it will work, while doing the actions that contribute to weight loss and you will overcome any and all barriers to the success you intend.

Yes, to diet correctly, you're going to pay a lot of attention to the food you put in your body. But there is an action far more important than that – making the decision to lose weight and deciding that you will maintain the weight loss. Then having someone who offers encouragement, and instills discipline during your weak moments, and validates you when you get results. You need a cheerleader and sometimes a coach who can deliver a good pep talk. I became this person for my husband and continued on to helping many others lose weight. In addition to those actions, I decided to also do everything I told him to do, "walking the walk" instead of merely "talking the talk". I lost 20 pounds along with him. So find someone who will be this person for you, better yet, who will do this diet with you. If they do not want to diet themselves, have them read this book and apply its principles to you.

The power of two can be more powerful than the power of one.

There are Abbi's Way Diet Coaches that can get you to where you want to go if you can't find someone to help.

The first step is deciding that you're going to help yourself and/or another lose weight while eating healthier, more nourishing food. This decision can have no doubts or reservations. In my case, I wanted to ensure my husband didn't have a heart attack or another non-optimum health condition. So my purpose, most definitely, didn't have any doubts or reservations. My necessity to make him healthier was very high. I got him to agree with my viewpoint. And discovered he shared the same purpose and necessity I did to get healthy fast but needed my help.

The second step is to create a plan and keep it simple. The answers to these five questions is your plan:

1. What is my purpose for this diet?

2. How much weight do I want to lose?

3. By what date do I want to lose the total weight?

5. What will I eat on my cheat days?

Now your plan is done and you are ready to begin the mechanics of losing weight fast and maintaining your intended ideal weight.

Important to note, you don't need luck on this program. Just do the program, as written in this book, and your ideal weight is inevitable.

You are now armed with the natural laws of how to effectively control your weight. You are already winning the game. Now go win a lot more!

APPENDIX

MORE CLIENT RESULTS

"About 8 weeks ago, I begin Abbi's Way eating plan. I have currently lost 30 lbs and I'm now at my lowest weight, in at least, the last 15 years.

This loss has been awesome but the most surprising elements of this plan are that I have seldom felt hungry and due to the fact that there is a "cheat day" built in, I have far fewer cravings because I know I will be able to 'scratch that itch'. And when I do cheat, I am not mentally beating myself up. I find that I am much better at controlling how much of the cheat I devour.

"I think I can honestly say that I am more alert and much less sluggish later in the evenings. I feel much better about myself because I know that I am eating more healthy foods and I'm changing my eating habits to a much more healthy lifestyle which will better me in the long run.

"This has been the easiest weight loss plan I have ever done and I also have a much higher certainty that I will be able to keep the weight off once I hit my final target. In fact, I believe that I am actually at the point in this plan that I really don't feel like I am on an eating plan anymore – it is really beginning to feel like my normal eating plan now. Thanks Abbi!" – Abbi's Way Client, Kevin C.

"For years, I have been looking for a way to be in better control of my body and my diet. There were short-term solutions but nothing ever worked with a high degree of success where I felt I could sustain the gains. The best part of Abbi's program was that it was simple to follow, it never left me hungry or agitated, and it followed the basic laws of weight loss. She kept me winning and more importantly allowed me to celebrate my success along the way, which kept me motivated to keep progressing.

Abbi's program gets your attitude toward your body and food straight first which then led me to easily follow the program. I lost 40 lbs in 10-12 weeks and I did it naturally and healthy. Do it!"– Abbi's Way Client, Eric M.

"Up until I started Abbi's Way, I had always felt like I was fighting a losing battle with my weight. I think I had done weight watchers at least 4 times since I was 18 and while I would lose weight, it was an awful struggle and the results were never consistent no matter how well I followed the program. And it would take, what felt like forever, to lose a few pounds, so I didn't easily see the results. About 10 years ago, I got tired of fighting and gave up. I gained a whopping 70+ pounds. That weight gain resulted in me giving up a lot of other things but I mostly lost my love for life and being social. I hated going out, I had headaches all the time, I was tired every afternoon, I didn't sleep well, and I was miserable with myself. I knew I needed to confront it and lose the weight but the thought of weight watchers or some other fad diet wasn't appealing to me. And then Abbi called...

"Abbi's diet is exactly what I was looking for and IT WORKS! I can see the difference and so can my family! I have lost over ten pounds, per month, since starting and I now have something that is guaranteed to help me lose weight. Two HUGE differences in this plan vs. any others: (1.) I have someone there for me. Abbi has worked with me and helped me stay on track even with traveling and major family events five out of the last eleven weeks...I could NEVER have said that with any other program I have been on, (2.) I get a cheat day. This one is big for me and I can see how before, when going off plan I would completely give up and have to work twice as hard to get back on because I saw it as a failure. Now, with a cheat day, I am able to take control and plan a day that I will cheat and start thinking about what it is I really want. It has made a huge difference.

"I can actually see myself achieving my goal weight and can even tell you an approximate date I will achieve it. My whole family has noticed the difference and is encouraging me in my quest; my husband is even getting into it and has lost some weight, which is great since diabetes runs rampant in his family. I cannot say enough about this program and I will be honest with you – I was not a believer when I started. All those other diets had turned me off. But, I now realize, this isn't a diet but a new way of life. It is the way to living a much cleaner and happier life. And believe me, I am so much happier eating Abbi's Way". – Abbi's Way Client, Dee B.

"Abbi's Way has given me an increased awareness of how what I put into my body can affect my overall well-being! I very quickly lost the 'bloat' that I was carrying around and I felt invigorated almost immediately as my body used the nutritious foods that I was giving it. My energy levels have definitely improved and I feel 10 years younger!

"My thoughts are more clear and concise - I don't feel 'foggy' or lethargic like I did prior to starting Abbi's program. I have better control in making decisions about what I want to eat and I am enjoying what I eat more than I have in a long time. I don't feel like I'm deprived of anything.
"This lifestyle change has made me feel so good about myself that it will easily become my new permanent existence! Thank you Abbi!!" – Abbi's Way Client, Jeanine M.

"I hope it's not health-related" that is the comment that usually follows, "Wow, you've lost weight..." when people see me.

"My response, 'It's absolutely health-related! We got sick and tired of being overweight!'

"My husband and I have been on Abbi's Way program for 2 ½ months and I have lost over 20 pounds. As a 'yo-yo dieter', I have tried every program imaginable over the years and Abbi's Way is the easiest, most manageable program I have ever used. No crazy foods, calorie counting, expensive supplements. It is more of a lifestyle change that I will continue to fall back on, even after I reach my goal.

"The 'Cheat Day' is a game-changer! It is so much easier to stick to the plan, knowing that my favorite foods are only a few days away.

"I took a girlfriend trip that was 5 straight cheat days, where I only gained 1.5 lbs. that were gone— and then some, only 3 days back on the plan. I feel I can enjoy a vacation without guilt, confident that I will quickly be back on track when I return.

"While I have 10 pounds left to reach my goal, I have no more 'try-on' clothes left in my closet, and it is actually a joy knowing that I will be comfortable in anything I pull out to wear. I have more energy, I sleep better, and I have more self-confidence.

"Abbi has been a great resource, and Abbi's Way has been the tool I needed to take my healthy life back under my control!" – Abbi's Way Client, Mary C.

"I am doing well on the diet. The biggest realization is being in control against urges and bad habits. This is key.

"I focus on what I can have and create on that, instead of being focused on the restrictions of what I can't have. My approach on the items, not part of this diet, is I don't want them due to the unwanted results. I feel much more at cause over my body". – Abbi's Way Client, Award Winning Executive Chef Z

THE AUTHOR'S GLOSSARY

Amino acids – the basic building blocks of protein. They are a vital part of your diet. Food consumed with amino acids, like eggs, will usually give you a burst of energy.

Antibodies – a protein that is a natural part of your immune system, which plays a function of fighting unwanted bacteria in the body and eliminating viruses.

Apathetic – an attitude that nothing can be done about anything.

Appetite – your desire or lack of desire for food. For instance, if you were hungry, you would have a strong appetite; if you're weren't hungry, you have lost your appetite.

Attitude – is a way of looking at something and how you act with that viewpoint. Someone who has a good attitude, working with others, is cooperative and in good coordination.

Biblical – in accordance with the Bible.

Binge – to do a lot of something excessively.

Body fat % – simply the percentage of fat your body holds. There is a certain amount of good fat a body must have to be in a healthy, optimum condition. When body fat goes into non-optimum ranges, health issues can ensue.

Bulldozer of Must Dos – a humorous phrase which communicates the enforcement of what must be done to achieve a result.

Burn – to use up.

Calorie – a unit of measured energy in food.

Carbs – short for carbohydrates. These are vital structural components of living cells. They are an important source of energy for the body.

Cheat day – also known as Stage Three of the Abbi's Way program. It is when you eat whatever you want, especially foods with more sugar and carbs

Cholesterol – a natural substance found in animal tissue that helps support the health of a human body. Too much cholesterol can be an issue when there is a high concentration of it. A high concentration can block arteries, leading to heart problems.

Client – a person who has paid for a service and/or product.

Come hell or high water – a phrase that communicates getting something done, in spite of all barriers.

Curbing – to check and keep something in control.

Deprivation – a state in which something is kept away from someone.

Diet – the chosen food and drink consumed by a person. When a person says they're going on a diet, they usually mean they are choosing food and drink that help them lose and or maintain their body weight.

Dismay – an emotional state of disappointment.

Enzymes – proteins created by cells. They break down starch, fat and help with digesting other proteins. They are important to the health of the human body.

Fat – 1. an abundance of body flesh 2. body tissue that serves as a source of energy for a healthy body.

GMO – an abbreviation for - genetically modified organism. This simply means that the DNA of something has been genetically altered to change the genes normally found in that entity.

Grinchy Claus – a name in reference to the Grinch Who Stole Christmas.

Hormones – found in all living organisms. As part of the human body, they send vital signals throughout the body to perform survival functions such as childbirth, when to eat, etc.

Ketosis – a natural process in the body that burns fat. This process can be increased or decreased depending upon what is consumed in one's diet.

Lb – a unit of body weight.

LDL – an abbreviation for "low-density lipoprotein". This is a type of cholesterol, consisting of protein and fat (lipo) in the human body that helps keep a health heart. Too much of it is not good for the health of the heart.

Legumes – plants that bear their fruit in pods, etc. Peas and beans are examples. They are low in fat and high protein.

Maintenance – the activity of keeping something in the desired condition or state intended.

Metabolism – the combination of several functions of the human body that use food, etc. to create the energy for living. It is known that a high rate of metabolism can burn fat faster and result in weight loss. A slower rate of metabolism can conserve energy and burn less fat.

Metabolize – the action of the body taking calories and putting them to healthy use of the body.

Mr. & Mrs Jekyll and Hyde – a humorous reference to a person marked by two personalities - one being nice and the other being mean.

Muscle – body tissue that consists of cells that contract and produce changing motion.

Obese – is a condition in which your body fat content begins to threaten your physical health. In other words, the body holds an excessive amount of fat.

Organ – a part of the body that performs a specific function to contribute to the overall physical health of an individual.

Plus-point – something that is a positive aspect of something.

Portion –an intended, specific amount of something. For instance, a specific amount of food one intends to eat.

Protein – a substance, found in fish, meat, eggs, etc., that is vital to the health of the human body. The original meaning of the word is Greek in origin and meant – first.

Resounding – clearly and emphatically so.

Result – that which occurs as a consequence of some action or actions.

Self-conscious – aware and uncomfortable with yourself. For instance, a self-conscious person may not be happy with how they look or how they talk.

Soap opera – dramatic, everyday events that are usually sensationalized for television or radio to entertain an audience.

Stage One – this is the stage of the Abbi's Way program that is for the intended weight loss of the client. It is a very specific program of actions.

Stage Two – this is the stage of Abbi's Way program that is to ensure the intended, ideal weight is maintained over a the desired amount of time. It is a very specific program of actions

Stage Three – this stage is the "cheat day". This is where you eat anything you want, including foods with higher sugar content (if desired). As part of the program, there are Stage Three days you take while progressing on Stage One or Stage Two on Abbi's Way.

Sugar – a crystal like substance used as a sweetener and a preservative in food, etc. It is a carbohydrate and too much of it can cause minor and major health issues with body.

Supersizing – to change something to a much larger size.

Supplement – something added. For instance, something added to your regular diet to better improve your health, such as JuicePlus+.

Synthetic – something made from artificial materials or substances that is not natural.

'tis nobler... – a reference to Shakespeare's story of Hamlet when he was wavering between two different extremes and could not make a decision.

Validating – to confirm the rightness of something and make it more real to self and/or others.

Veggies – short for vegetables. Edible items derived from plants.

Weight – a measurement of the body's mass.

Weight Management – effective daily control of the body, and what is put into it, to maintain the intended desired weight.

Who's mouthses – a humorous reference to the Whos of the story, How the Grinch Stole Christmas, by Dr Seuss. These were tiny creatures that lived in Whoville and who had very small mouths.

Win – something you intended to do and did or something you intended to not do and didn't. For instance, if intended to lose five pounds within 6 days and did so, it is a "win". If you intended to not eat ice cream one evening and didn't, it is another "win".

Winning – a continuous state of getting what you intend in life. Or not getting what you don't intend in life.

Water % – the content of water in the tissues, the blood, the bones and elsewhere in the body. This makes up a significant portion of the human body. It is important to the health of the body to have the right amount of water.

Wonka's Chocolate River of Bliss – a humorous reference to the drinkable, chocolate river as shown in the classic movie, Willy Wonka's Chocolate Factory.

FOR A FREE DIET CONSULTATION

EMAIL

ABBISWAYDIET@GMAIL.COM